CBD OIL CANN,

PAIN

The Beginner's Guide to Hemp Oil
and CBD Cannabidiol for Pain Relief
from Arthritis and Inflammation,
Eliminate Acne & Improve Skin for
Better Health

By

Andrew Page

Copyright @2018

TABLE OF CONTENT

INTRODUCTION

It's a frightening statistic: more than 20% of the adult population in the United States suffers from chronic pain. This statistic is troubling because it proves that a large number of people are suffering from chronic pain. However - if you do not want to be part of this statistic, pay attention to the content of this guide.

If you ask this 20 % of adults suffering from this problem, they'll tell you that it can and does happen. And they'll also tell you the best thing you can do is to learn the best way to get relief from your pain. That's the whole essence of this book.

In just moments you'll find out how to use CBD oil to get relief from pain. Read on...

Specifically, you will discover:

- What CBD is and how it works

- How it provides pain relief from various health issues

- How to use hemp oil on your skin

- Precautions, side effects, and risks of hemp oil

4

CHAPTER 1

WHAT IS CBD AND HOW DOES IT WORK?

What is CBD?

While the two most active compounds in the cannabis sativa plant are cannabidiol (CBD) and tetrahydrocannabinol (THC), THC is the most popular because its psychoactive properties make it highly intoxicating when consumed.

But despite its non-psychoactive properties, CBD has many health benefits. However, products from the cannabis plant are subjected to legal laws. Hence, be sure your state of residence legalizes the use of cannabis products.

How CBD works

Phyto (plant-produced) and endo (produced by the body naturally) cannabinoids are the two types of cannabinoids. An example of the phytocannabinoid is the CBD.

Phytocannabinoids and endocannabinoids are similar in action. Hence, phytocannabinoids can supplement what's being produced by the endocannabinoids in the body.

Your body's immune, nervous, reproductive and digestive systems have receptors for cannabinoids.

Though cannabinoids can influence the functions of your body's mitochondria and neurotransmitters, control metabolism and reduce inflammation in your body, they cant cure all health issues in your body despite being able to interact with almost all body systems.

The best way to start using CBD oil is to take its capsules or orally ingest the oil. If your migraine is severe and you're at home, consider vaping the oil. According to the national cancer institute (NCI), this method of ingestion is faster than other methods because it delivers the oil into your bloodstream immediately you vape it.

Though there are currently no rules for CBD oil dosage for migraine, you can start with 2.5mg CBD oil dosage per day to relieve your chronic pain. Then, increase it up to 20 mg per day. Thus, you will get accustomed to the oil and make you less susceptible to any side effects.

10

CHAPTER 2

USE OF HEMP OIL AND CBD CANNABIDIOL FOR PAIN RELIEF

Here are the top four benefits of Hemp oil:

1. Relief from Chronic Pain

The use of marijuana for relieving pain dates back to 2900 BC. However, recent scientific research has proven that the CBD component in marijuana is responsible for pain relief. Four of the functions controlled by the endocannabinoid system of your human body are immune system response, pain, appetite, and sleep. These endocannabinoids are neurotransmitters which can bind to your nervous system through the cannabinoid receptors.

Research has proven that CBD relieves pain through its interaction with your body's neurotransmitters, decreasing inflammation and improving the activities of the endocannabinoid receptors.

Oral CBD treatment on some rats with chronic pain decreased not just the pain but the inflammation. Similarly, CBD injections on another group of rats with chronic pain decreased their pain response to the injection.

New evidence suggests that humans with pain from arthritis and multiple sclerosis can be effectively treated with a combination of cannabidiol (CBD) and tetrahydrocannabinol (THC) without intoxicating them. Pain from multiple sclerosis can now be treated with Sativex (an oral spray that combines THC and CBD)

When 45 people were subjected to Savitex for four weeks, they were able to start walking with less pain and without muscle spasms. Also, fifty-seven people with arthritis had more quality sleep and didn't experience pain during their movements or when resting after they took Savitex for one month.

2. Eliminate Acne

With more than 9% of the population suffering from this skin condition, acne can be classified as common skin trouble. Top four factors that can cause acne are the overproduction of sebum (the sebaceous glands in the skin generates this oily secretion), an underlying inflammation, bacteria, and genetics.

Recent research has shown that CBD oil's anti-inflammatory properties and its ability to decrease sebum production may help to treat acne.

CBD oil eliminates acne by:

- Preventing the activation of inflammatory cytokines and other 'pro-acne' agents,

- Inhibiting the sebaceous glands from generating excess sebum and

- Exerting anti-inflammatory actions

However, there is still ongoing research on the use of CBD oil for the treatment of acne.

3. Relief from Gout

Gout is a type of arthritis caused by excess uric acid in your joints (especially your big toe) leading to pain and inflammation. Gouts can also be precursors to kidney stones because some of the uric acids can combine over time to cause kidney stones.

Heat, pain, redness, and swelling are the top symptoms of gout.

CBD oil can provide you relief from gout because it boosts the endocannabinoid 2-ag to attach with the cb2 receptor of your body immune system. This prevents the cb2 receptor from generating attack cells that are causing the inflammation.

4. Improve Skin Health

Whether by oral ingestion or in mixture with your lotion, CBD oil or hemp seed oil can be highly beneficial to your skin.

- **Balances out oily skin**

Without clogging your skin pores, hemp oil can moisturize your skin regardless of its type. By moderating and hydrating your skin's oil production, it can provide a balance for your oily skin.

Skin dryness can also induce acne since it can cause your skin to produce oil in excess. Hemp oil reduces acne in dry skin in the same way as oily skin.

- ***Calms inflammation and irritation on the skin***

Gamma-linolenic acid (GLA) is one of the omega-6 fatty acids in hemp oil. When applied properly, it simultaneously encourages skin growth, promotes new cell generation and acts as a strong anti-inflammatory agent.

Hence, it helps to keep your skin nourished and moisturized while decreasing symptoms of acne, psoriasis and any other skin issues.

- **Provides treatment for atopic eczema**

The abundance of omega-6 and omega-3 fatty acids in your skin can significantly reduce symptoms of atopic eczema. And since hemp seed oil contains large amounts of omega-6 and omega-3 fatty acids, it is effectively useful for the treatment of this skin condition.

- **Anti-aging attributes**

Hemp oil contains large concentrations of linoleic acids and oleic acids which play an important part in anti-aging and skin health, but can't be produced by the body. Hemp oil inhibits the development of aging while reducing fine lines and wrinkles.

For the best results, you need to

add the hemp oil to your diet.

5. Boosts hair growth

By supplying your skin with keratin, omega 3, omega 6 and omega nine fatty acids, hemp oil:

- Boosts your hair growth

- Helps with the blood circulation to ensure the hair follicles can support the growth.

- Helps your hair to maintain its natural texture

Apart from moisturizing your skin and hair, hemp oil also prevents water loss.

Other Health Applications of Hemp Oil

1. Lowering High Blood Pressure

Metabolic syndrome, heart attack, and stroke are health conditions associated with high blood pressure. If you have undergone stress that can increase your blood pressure, a single dose of CBD can lower your blood pressure. CBD can lower blood pressure because it contains stress-reducing and anxiety-reducing properties.

Also, since it has a strong antioxidant and stress-reducing properties, it can decrease inflammation and death of cells associated with heart disease.

2. Reducing Psychotic Symptoms

If you are suffering from mental disorders such as schizophrenia, CBD is proven to reduce the symptoms of these disorders.

3. **Prevent the spread of tumor effects either in the lung, colon, brain, prostate or breast**

4. **Prevention of diabetes and reduction of inflammation**

5. **Heal those addicted to psychostimulants, opioid, cocaine, tobacco, and cannabis.**

It may even reduce the intoxicating effects of THC in the body.

6. It provides pain relief from inflammation.

CBD protects your body from attacking itself by inhibiting production of cytokine and stimulating t-regulatory cells.

CHAPTER 3

HOW TO USE HEMP OIL ON YOUR SKIN

There are two main ways to apply hemp oil on your skin:

- Direct application on your skin
- Oral ingestion

1. *Direct (Topical) Application on Your Skin Via Creams And Lotions*

If there are dry patches on your skin, you can soothe them quickly by applying the hemp oil directly on your skin. However, to prevent an undesired reaction, perform a patch test before using the oil.

You can perform a patch test by following these steps:

- Wash and dry a small part of the affected area

- Apply a small quantity of the pure hemp oil

- Cover with a dry bandage for 24 hours

Should you experience any irritation such as itching, burning, and redness, you shouldn't be using the oil; you are sensitive to it.

Remove the bandage at any time you experience irritation within 24 hours; wash the area with soap and water. However, if you don't suffer any irritation, apply the oil to every affected part and wash with warm after two minutes.

You can mix the hemp oil with soothing and anti-inflammatory ingredients in the following proportions:

- $\frac{1}{2}$ cup hemp oil

- 4 teaspoons melted coconut oil

- 8 drops rosemary oil or any other skin-boosting essential oil such as lavender oil

Pro tip: most essential oils are toxic, so don't use them orally. Rather, you should mix them with other oils before applying them directly on your skin.

2. Oral Ingestion

Oral ingestion of hemp oil provides the same benefits as a direct application on the skin. While you may experience slight digestive disturbance through oral consumption of hemp oil. But you are not likely to experience any skin irritation.

Don't take hemp oil orally without consulting your doctor. Hemp seeds can inhibit platelets because they can interact with blood thinners. Once your doctor approves, you can consume two daily teaspoons in two doses or at once.

Other options you can use to consume hemp oil is by using it to cook or stirring it in your soup, salad dressings, smoothies, and other foods.

CBD is also available in the following forms:

- Teas
- Vape pens/oils
- Tinctures
- Oils
- Edibles

CHAPTER 4

PRECAUTIONS, SIDE EFFECTS, AND RISKS OF HEMP OIL

Hemp oil doesn't have any psychoactive properties or have any THC. Hence, it is safe for most people. However, one major precaution you can take is to start with small quantities of hemp oil (such as two teaspoons per day) to prevent loose stools or digestive troubles

If you consume the wrong dosage, you may experience any of these mild side effects which should disappear within four hours:

- Bloating

- Diarrhea

- Vomiting

- Dry mouth

- Nausea

CONCLUSION

Regardless of the mode of application, there are a lot of benefits associated with hemp oil. It is effective for your skin health, and there have been no reported cases on any side effects. New health benefits of CBD oil is sure to be discovered because there is ongoing research on its benefits.

However, based on current research, it remains a strong and effective treatment for a lot of health issues. Even if you have no health issues, you can supplement your diet with CBD oil to maintain an overall healthy lifestyle.

One important reason why you need to consult your doctor before consuming CBD oil is that the safety and effectiveness of most CBD products cannot be guaranteed since they are mostly unregulated.

Don't pack away this information in your noggin, it won't do you any good. Take action today by buying your CBD oil to get relief from your pain very quickly.

Regardless of the mode of application, there are a lot of benefits associated with hemp oil. It is effective for your skin health, and there have been no reported cases on any side effects. New health benefits of CBD oil is sure to be discovered because there is ongoing research on its benefits.

However, based on current research, it remains a strong and effective treatment for a lot of health issues. Even if you have no health issues, you can supplement your diet with CBD oil to maintain an overall healthy lifestyle.

One important reason why you need to consult your doctor before consuming CBD oil is that the safety and effectiveness of most CBD products cannot be guaranteed since they are mostly unregulated.

Don't pack away this information in your noggin, it won't do you any good. Take action today by buying your CBD oil to get relief from your pain very quickly.

THANK YOU FOR

READING TILL

THE END

REFERENCES

https://highlandpharms.com/cbd-hemp-oil/

https://www.greenrelief.ca/blog/cbd-oil-cannabis-vs-hemp-difference/

https://www.mydomaine.com/what-is-cbd-oil

https://www.medicalnewstoday.com/articles/319796.php

CPSIA information can be obtained
at www.ICGtesting.com
Printed in the USA
LVHW081326220819
628587LV00016B/572/P

9 781730 905926